AF431604

Essential Oils for Beginners

Natural Remedies for Health and Beauty

Catalina Morris

iv

© Text Copyright 2022 by Catalina Morris - All rights reserved.

Table of Contents

Introduction..1

CHAPTER ONE

What Are Essential Oils? 3

What Are Essential Oils for? 3

What Are the Benefits of Using Essential Oils?........................5

The Origins and History of Essential Oils 6

How Are Essential Oils Made?...7

Steam Distillation 8

Water Distillation 9

Cold Press Extraction..10

Maceration...10

Enfleurage..11

CHAPTER TWO

How to Use and Store Essential Oils....................................13

Inhalation 13

Direct Skin Contact...16

Diluted Skin Contact...17

Buying and Storing Essential Oils...18

Oxygen...19

Heat and Moisture 20

Light...20

Safety 21

CHAPTER THREE

How to Blend Essential Oils..23

Carrier Oils 23

Mixing Essential Oils 25

vi

CHAPTER FOUR

Common Essential Oils 30

    Bergamot 30
    Cinnamon 30
    Chamomile 31
    Clove.. 31
    Eucalyptus 31
    Frankincense.. 31
    Grapefruit 32
    Geranium 32
    Jasmine 32
    Lavender 33
    Lemon... 33
    Mint 34
    Oregano 34
    Peppermint.. 34
    Rose 34
    Rosemary 35
    Sandalwood 35
    Sweet Orange.. 35
    Tea Tree 35
    Ylang-Ylang 35

CHAPTER FIVE

Essential Oil Blends for Skin Care.................................... 37

    Stretch Mark Reducing Blend 37
    Scar Salve 37
    Whipped Eczema Cream 38
    Whipped Body Butter.. 39
    Wrinkle Cream 39
    Natural Toner.. 40
    Oil Blend for Age Spots 40
    Sweet Sugar Scrub... 41

Bath Bomb for Skin Care 41

CHAPTER SIX

Essential Oil Recipes for Acne..44

Easy Acne Recipe 44
Blackheads Begone..44
Pimple Pop Roller 45
Acne Treatment Cream 45
Herbal Face Scrub for Acne 46

CHAPTER SEVEN

Essential Oil Blends for Hair Care..47

Itchy Scalp Remedy 47
Anti-Dandruff Shampoo 47
Dry Scalp Cure 48
Deep Hair Conditioner..48
Hair Moisturizer..49
Beard Oil Recipe..50
DIY Lice Treatment..50

CHAPTER EIGHT

Essential Oil Blends for Stress Relief.....................................52

Soothing Blend for Anxiety..52
Relaxing Blend for Stress Relief 53
Stress Relieving Bath..54
Lavender Remedy for Insomnia 54
Sleepy Time Bath 55
Quick Relaxation 55
Calm a Child 56

CHAPTER NINE

Essential Oil Blends for Pain Relief.......................................57

Quick Relief Blend for Arthritis..57

Migraine Remedy 57
Aromatherapy Bath for Migraines................................. 58
Muscle Relaxer 58
Soothing Bath for Muscle Tension................................ 59
Basic Pain Relief Salve 59

CHAPTER TEN

Essential Oil Recipes for Allergies and Sunburn........................ 61

Allergy Relief.. 61
Allergy Relief Bath.. 61
Poison Ivy Treatment 62
Essential Oil Remedy for Sunburn 62

CHAPTER ELEVEN

Essential Oil Blends for the Home 64

Air Freshener Blend 64
Disinfectant Blend 64
Cleaning Scrub 65
Natural Pest Repellent 66

Conclusion 67

Introduction

Essential oils are an age-old method of healing the mind and body through our sense of smell and the power of nature. Many plants have healing properties. For example, echinacea is an immune booster, and chamomile relaxes and rejuvenates the body. We frequently use plants in medicine and often brew teas and herbal infusions. But sometimes, that is not an option, be that from a lack of fresh plants or certain properties that make many healing plants unsuitable for ingestion. This is when we turn to essential oils.

Essential oils are harvested from sweet-smelling plants. They are highly concentrated liquids that contain strong scents representing the plants they come from. Essential oils have been used for thousands of years around the world for the holistic treatment of health problems. Today, essential oils are again gaining popularity as consumers discover the many great benefits that these oils provide.

Using essential oils for healing isn't as simple as buying whatever smells best and sniffing a few drops each day. Not all oils have the same effects, and they can't all be used in the same way. You may combine oils that counter each other, or you may be applying an essential oil in the wrong place or in a situation where it won't be as effective as it could be. This book is here to help guide you through the basics of using essential oils, from how essential oils work and where they come from, to techniques and recipes to blend and create your own essential oil products to suit your lifestyle and preferences.

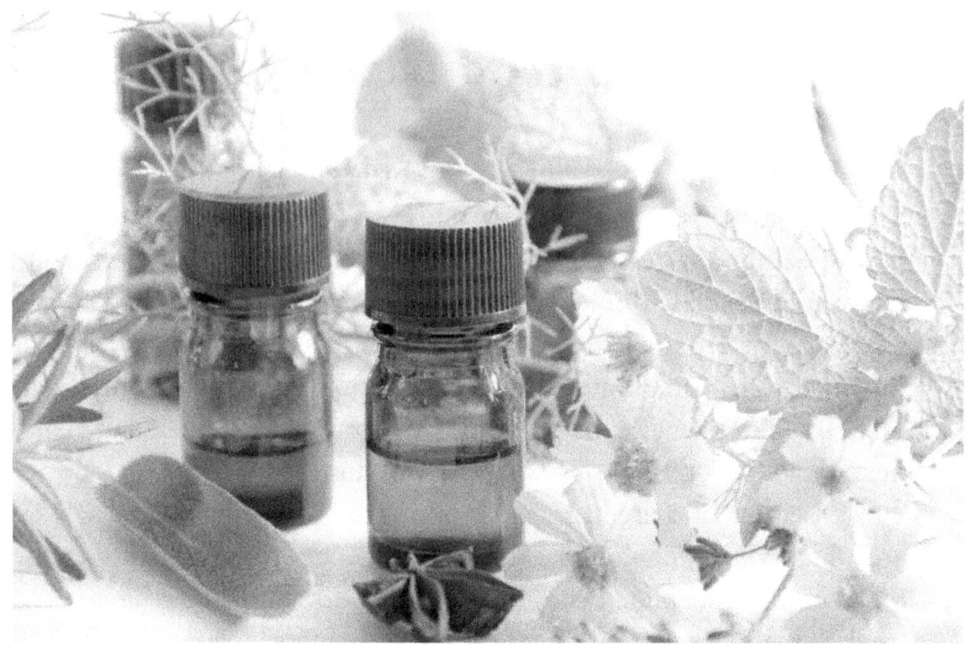

CHAPTER ONE

What Are Essential Oils?

Essential oils are concentrated substances extracted from plants, which maintain the smell and taste of said plant—i.e., its *essence.* These oils come in various forms and are commonly used in products such as lotions, beard oils, etc. There are hundreds of different essential oils, each with its characteristics. Even oils extracted from the same plant can vary from each other, depending on the extraction process, the initial condition of the plant, how pure and concentrated the oil is, and many other elements that make these oils unique.

Essential oils are usually mixed with a carrier oil and sold in stores. Essential oils are very easy to come by and are commonly found in drugstores, apothecaries, and natural health stores. Some essential oils may be more expensive than others, depending on the rarity of the plant and the difficulty of extracting the oils from the plant.

What Are Essential Oils for?

Essential oils are widely used in *aromatherapy.* Aromatherapy is a process through which specific scents are inhaled through the nose, which then interact with the chemicals inside the brain to induce positive, healing effects within your mind and body. The aromas are most commonly released into the air through scented candles, in which essential oils are used during the manufacturing process. Aromatherapy is often combined with other forms of health and relaxation treatments, such as massages. In these cases, essential oils are added to the oils and lotions used in the massage. Aromatherapy can also be used more casually, such as tucking a sachet filled with herbs and essential oils of relaxing properties under your pillow to help you sleep, or placing a bowl of potpourri in your workspace with some rejuvenating essential oils to give you a little extra energy to get you through the day.

Essential oils can also be mixed with lotions, beard oils, and various skin creams and treatments. Not only will this have similar effects to that of aromatherapy, but many of the plant chemicals within the oils will be absorbed into the skin. These chemicals are nourishing and helpful for your body and skin. Specific combinations of lotions and certain essential oils can be used as moisturizers that work exceptionally well with dry skin, or as night creams that help relax the mind and body.

Another use for essential oils is simply making spaces and objects smell nice. Besides the many benefits different essential oils can have on your mind and body, these oils usually smell great. You can use your favorite scents all over the house to create a lovely, fresh environment. A good example is to put a few drops of your favorite essential oil on the inside of a roll of toilet paper, which will keep your bathroom smelling lovely, or add a few drops of oil on a piece of cloth to keep in your shoe closet, to eliminate any unwanted odors.

Many would argue that you can use the plant itself rather than its essential oil, which might be cheaper, especially if you have that plant growing in your garden. The first and most important reason this may not necessarily be accurate is that the essential oils are concentrated, making their smell and effects on your body much more potent than when using the plant itself, whether fresh or dry. Furthermore, some plants are very difficult to come by and are seasonal, meaning you are limiting any benefits to the period in which the plant grows abundantly. You are further limited to the plants that grow in your climate, and the plants you use will eventually dry out, often losing their smell and healing properties. Lastly, essential oils are more convenient to use, as they can be easily mixed with other products or objects. It's easier and more pleasant to mix a few drops of lavender oil in your body cream than to rub crushed lavender leaves and flowers all over your body.

One thing you must keep in mind is that essential oils are not meant to be ingested. Some plants, such as vanilla and lemon, go through a different process to develop a concentrated extract of their flavor for use in cooking and baking. Still, these are extracts and are fairly different from essential oils.

What Are the Benefits of Using Essential Oils?

Other than being convenient and completely natural, essential oils provide health benefits that can improve the quality of your life.

Among the ailments treated with essential oils, stress and anxiety are the most common. Several studies have proven that certain essential oils can relieve stress and relax the body, especially when combined with physical therapy, such as massage and yoga.

As shown in Chapter 9, essential oils can be used to treat headaches, be they only a minor irritation or a severe migraine. Not only are the scents soothing and comforting, but the minerals and vitamins found in certain plant oils are great for treating underlying problems of headaches. Simply rub a few drops of lavender or mint oil onto your forehead and temples, and you will feel relief almost instantly.

Many plants, such as peppermint and tea tree, act as antibiotics, while others, like rosemary, can reduce inflammation. The essential oils of these plants contain potent properties since they are concentrated and can be applied directly to affected areas. Applying specific essential oils to a wound may reduce swelling and prevent infection.

Essential oils may be used to overcome insomnia and help you enjoy a sound sleep. Many types of plants help relax the mind, and their oils can be used to create a peaceful atmosphere to help you fall asleep. On the other end of the spectrum, there are essential oils that can increase brain activity, invigorate the brain, and make you feel more energetic and ready for the day. It's important to keep these two types of oils apart, as using them together will cancel their effects and confuse your body.

The Origins and History of Essential Oils

Essential oils and their use for aromatherapy were initially discovered by the ancient Egyptians. This was the first civilization to cultivate plants purely for the purpose of extracting their oils. The oils were then used in cosmetics, medical rituals and procedures, and even the embalming process. These ancient people used a form of enfleurage to extract essential oils, using whatever types of fat were on hand. The biggest limitation they faced was that the kinds of essential oils available were limited to the plants that grew in the surrounding area. During the same period, eastern countries such as India and China began delving into the use of essential oils, which later became a prominent feature in both countries' medical practices.

As the ancient Greek culture began to develop, they picked up the use of essential oils from the Egyptians and used them as medical treatments. Even Hippocrates, the most renowned medical practitioner of that time, believed in the healing powers of essential oils and used them frequently with massages. Essential oils also gained a spiritual connection and were often used in religious ceremonies and rituals. In religious texts, such as the Bible, you will find the use of essential oils in certain situations mentioned quite often.

Next came the Roman Empire, which adopted many Greek uses and beliefs into their culture, including essential oils. The Romans continued to use essential oils in their medical practice. Because sanitation and cleanliness were important aspects of their daily lives, the Roman people often added fragrant essential oils to their bathwater for more rejuvenating, relaxing aromatic baths.

Shortly after the fall of the Roman Empire, during the middle ages, essential oils lost their purpose as a medical tool but were still a prominent part of religious practices. Because bathing wasn't widespread during those times, even among the nobility and upper classes, essential oils were instead employed to cover any bad odors.

During the Renaissance period, when people turned back to the knowledge of the ancient Greeks and Romans, the use of essential oils as a tool for healing gradually became popular again. Healers and doctors used essential oils more and more frequently until a famous French perfumer and chemist in the early twentieth century named Rene Maurice Gattefosse created the phrase *aromatherapy* and boosted the popularity of essential oils even more. In 1910, he burned his hand and poured distilled lavender oil over the wound in an attempt to ease the pain, as it was the nearest on hand. Not only did the lavender oil ease the pain better than expected, but further use of the oil proved to help prevent scarring and infection and help the burn heal. Gattefosse experimented with essential oils, which eventually led to aromatherapy becoming a significant part of treating injuries and infections on the battlefield during the second world war.

In the '70s and '80s, essential oils gained another boost in popularity through a general interest in natural remedies and healing techniques due to a desire to return to nature and protect the environment. Today, essential oils are not only a popular natural healing aide but also a great alternative to replacing harmful chemicals all over the home.

How Are Essential Oils Made?

Several methods are used to extract essential oils from plants, most of which are a form of distillation or pressing. Different methods are used depending on what is most effective for a particular plant and its various parts. For example, the best method for mint leaves may be ineffective for extracting oils from citrus peels or grape seeds. Here are a few basic methods that you can use to extract essential oils.

Steam Distillation

This is the most popular form of extraction—especially for commercial use. The entire plant, including the roots, leaves, stems, flowers, seeds, and peels, are put into a distillation machine. The apparatus containing the plant is placed over water, and the steam from that water breaks through the plant materials, extracting oils.

1. The plant material is placed inside a special container, usually made from stainless steel, often called the still. Steam is let into the still through an inlet on the bottom.

2. As the steam filters through the plant material, the natural oils and liquids within are heated and turned to vapor.

3. The vapor, which is slightly heavier than regular steam, is funneled to a separate container called a condenser, where the vapor is cooled and turned back into a liquid.

4. This liquid is then transferred into a separator. The liquid is a mixture of oil and water, but as those don't mix, they will be separated. The essential oil is then skimmed off the top of the water and transferred for packaging or to be worked into other products.

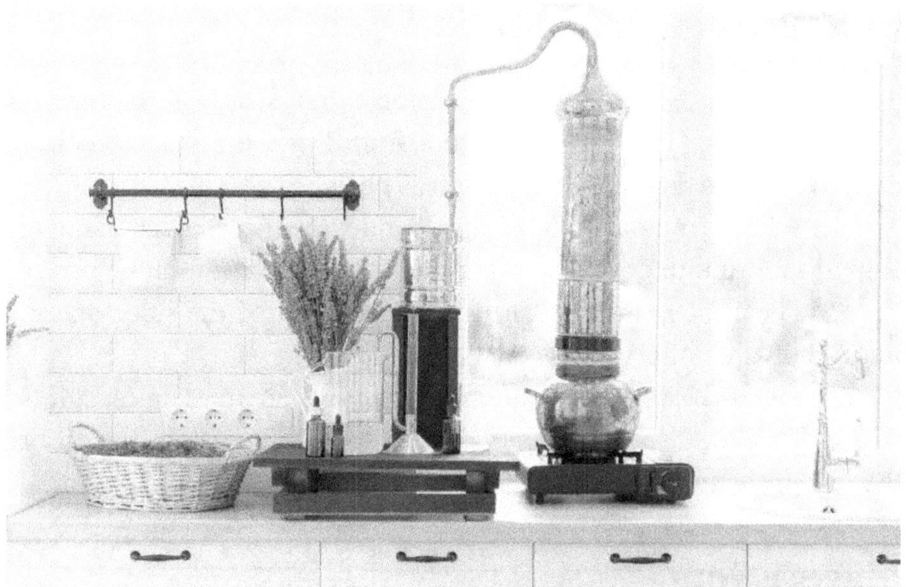

Water Distillation

This is similar to steam distillation but is used for more delicate plants such as orange blossom, which would clump and overheat if exposed to steam. Rather than using steam, the plant material is submerged in clean, purified water. The water is then heated to the boiling point until it becomes vapor. This vapor then goes through the same condensation and separation process as steam distillation. The water that is separated from the essential oil is usually infused with the smell, flavor, and some of the nutrients of the plant material and is often refined and sold as a product. A good example is rose water or orange blossom water. The main purpose of the water is to protect the essential oils extracted from being exposed to too much heat and burning, which causes a chemical reaction that will affect the properties of the final product.

Cold Press Extraction

This very intense method uses pressure to physically force the oils out of the plant. Typically used with fruit, this method is especially effective for extracting oils from citrus peels.

1. Whole fruits are placed inside a device that pierces the outer skin of the fruit, thus also piercing the oil sacks present in the peel.

2. The fruit is then crushed to squeeze all of the juice and oil out, which are collected in a container.

3. The juice and oil are filtered to remove any remaining solids.

4. The liquids are then moved to a separator to skim the oil off the rest of the juice.

Maceration

This process uses solvents—usually a form of carrier oil—to extract the scent, coloring, and healing chemicals from the plant. The product of this method is usually much more concentrated and potent than oils from the distillation process, as these carrier oils can extract some of the heavier compounds typically left behind during a distillation. This process requires that your plant product be as dry as possible, as moisture can encourage microbial growth, turning your oil rancid. A good way to prevent this is to add a small amount of wheat germ oil or vitamin E oil.

1. The dried plant material is chopped and ground into a coarse powder, and placed inside a sealable container.

2. The solvents are added, and the mixture is left for roughly a week while being shaken constantly. This lets the solvents begin absorbing the chemicals and oils of the plant material.

3. The mixture is strained, and the remaining solid plant material is pressed to extract any remaining oil.

4. The strained and pressed liquids are mixed and filtered until clear.

5. The base oil, which may have changed color during the maceration process, is now placed in a sealed container and stored in a cool, dry place for around twelve months.

Enfleurage

Although this technique isn't very common anymore, it is one of the oldest methods of extracting essential oils. It is also one of the easiest ways to extract essential oils without specialized equipment, despite being time-consuming. This technique uses odorless animal or plant fat that has been purified and is normally in a solid-state at room temperature. There are two different versions of this technique: cold enfleurage and hot enfleurage. Each follows the same process, but the fat is heated into a liquid form with hot enfleurage. This technique is most commonly used for flower-based material.

1. Odorless fat, usually tallow or lard, is spread over glass plates held in a chassis frame. In cold enfleurage, the fat is allowed to set, while in hot enfleurage, it is heated and kept in a liquid state.

2. Whole flowers or flower petals are lightly pressed into the fat and left for a few days to draw the scent and nutritional chemicals out of the plant and into the fat.

3. The flower petals are left in the fat until they have lost all their scents and oils are depleted. If the fat has not been infused to your liking, you can replace the depleted flowers or petals with new, fresh ones. Depending on the plant type and the intensity of the infusion, this process may take a few weeks or even months.

4. Once properly infused, the fat is washed with alcohol to remove the essential oils. The alcohol is kept in an open container, and as the alcohol dissolves, clean essential oil is left behind. The infused fat is usually used to make scented soaps.

There are a few more methods of extracting essential oils through the use of chemicals. These chemicals usually affect the natural state of the oils and the properties of the plants used, and are thus not considered methods of extracting natural essential oils.

CHAPTER TWO

How to Use and Store Essential Oils

Those who are intrigued by the benefits of essential oils might be a bit unsure about how to use them. You can enjoy the aromas and powers of these compounds in many different ways. Knowing how to use essential oils properly will maximize what they can do for you.

There are three main forms of exposing yourself to essential oils: inhalation, direct contact to your skin, and diluted contact. You should experiment a little to discover what works best for you.

Inhalation

As the name implies, this method consists of inhaling the scent of essential oil through the nose, letting the airborne particles of plant nutrients be absorbed into the body to begin their healing work. The simplest way to do this is to open a bottle of essential oil, hold it close to your nose, and take a deep breath. This allows you to inhale the scent directly, resulting in a strong effect from the oil. You should be careful with this method, for as effective as it is, it is also risky. First, the effect of the oil may be too strong and may cause headaches and lightheadedness. The oils from some plants, like cannabis, often have a drug-like effect on your body if you're exposed to large doses of concentrated oil too frequently, which can become harmful and addictive if not used carefully. Another problem with this method is that you risk exposing sensitive skin to undiluted oil. In their raw form, these oils can be hard on the skin and cause rashes, inflammation, and allergic reactions. This is not recommended if you are still new to the essential oil experience and are still deciding if you like using essential oils.

A safer form of this inhalation technique is through the aid of steam. You will need a bowl of warm water, a towel, a comfortable location, and most likely a small end table. First, find somewhere comfortable to set up, then heat the water to a temperature warm enough to create steam, but not warm enough that you will burn yourself. Add a few drops of your chosen essential oils to the water. Sit down on a comfortable surface (the edge of your bed, for example) and place the bowl of steaming water at a level where it's easy for you to bend over. Bend over the bowl with your face one to two hand-widths above the water's surface. Cover your head and the bowl with a towel and take your time to deeply inhale the rising steam, which carries vapors of the essential oils. The towel is used to keep the steam from dispersing too widely and weakening the healing effects of the oils.

The most common and often gentlest method of inhaling essential oils is the use of dispensers or diffusers. Dispensers are created to spread the scent of essential oils over a fairly large area, such as a whole room. The effect of the essential oil isn't as concentrated as with the previous two methods but can still work subtle changes on anyone who enters the range of the dispenser. There are various types of dispensers, such as ceramic, electric, sonic, and reed dispensers, that are specifically designed to use essential oils and can be bought in various stores. Candles can also be a type of dispenser, or you can make your own by adding a few drops of essential oil to your humidifier or simply placing a small, open container in front of an electric fan to spread the scent throughout the room. If you are considering using your humidifier, you should consult the manufacturer's manual, as not all humidifiers are suitable for the use of essential oils, and you may cause damage. You should also clean your humidifier often if using essential oils, and you should limit it to a fine mist. If placing a container in front of an electric fan, it will be more effective if both are placed high up, like up on the cupboard or the top shelf of your bookcase. You should also be careful of any accidental spillage and make sure the container is out of the reach of children or pets.

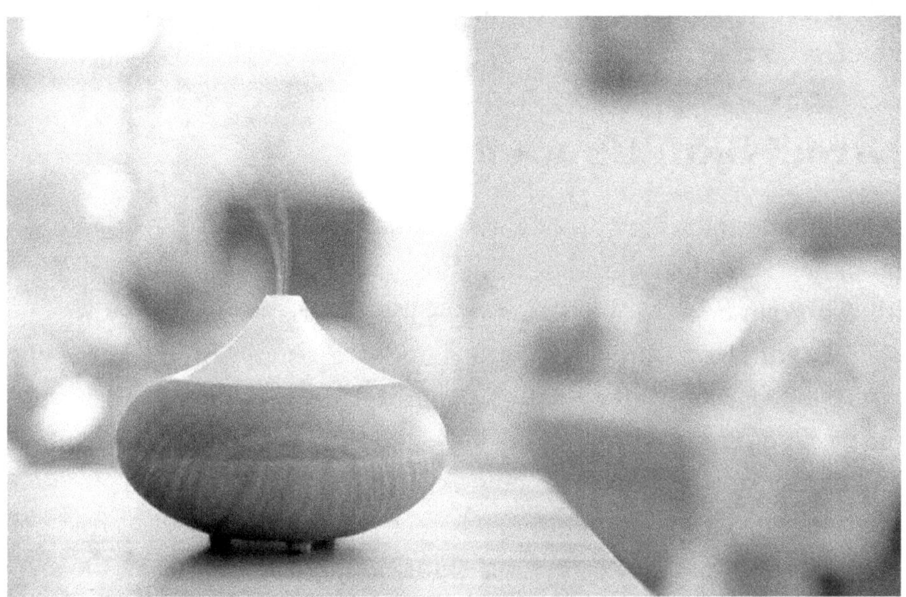

You may want the effect of a dispenser while still keeping the spread of the scent more personal. This is fairly easy to do and is called *dry evaporation.* This simple technique requires only a piece of dry material or a cotton ball. Add a few drops of essential oil to the material or cotton ball and hold it close to your face whenever you want to inhale the scent. You can keep the material in your purse or pocket to take it with you, or you can put a few drops of oil on the collar of your shirt. You can also place the scented material near the vents in your car to spread the scent inside. Adding a few drops of oil to your pillowcase is a great method to treat insomnia or stress. This technique uses the oil subtly and is very easy and convenient, especially since you can take it with you wherever you go. The biggest problem is that the scent will fade from the cloth or cotton ball, but you just need to add a few more drops whenever that happens.

When using any inhalation methods with essential oils, especially a dispenser, you need to consider those who share a living space with you, as your oils may affect them. Usually, there's no problem, but some essential oils can be harmful to small children, pregnant women, and pets.

Direct Skin Contact

Using essential oils directly on your skin allows your body to quickly absorb the vitamins, minerals, and other nutrients within the oil. This can be a great help but does have its risks.

Essential oils are very strong and are usually quite harsh for your skin. Because of this, you should always dilute your essential oil by blending it with a carrier oil—there will be more on blending and carrier oils in the next chapter.

Once your essential oil has been blended properly, you are ready to apply it directly to your skin. Simply rub the oil on the area of your body you want to affect, such as anti-inflammatory oils on a bruised, swollen spot or headache reducers on your forehead or temples. Oils with nourishing effects can be used over your entire body to help take care of your skin.

When applying essential oils directly to your skin, you should always keep the oil away from sensitive areas, such as the eyes or nose, to prevent irritation or pain. You should also be careful if your skin is sensitive in general, and you should consider any possible allergies. Always test your essential oils and carrier oils for allergies before using them in larger amounts. To do this, rub a small amount of the essential or carrier oil into a spot on the inside of your forearm, and leave it there for twenty-four hours. If your skin does not have any negative reactions such as itching, rashes, swelling, inflammation, or pain, your oils are safe to use. As long as you keep proper records, you can use this technique to test several oils at once, placing small dots of various oils in a line along the inside of your arm, from just below the elbow up to your wrist. Make sure you keep track of the types of oils you're testing and the order in which you applied them. If you are concerned about any reaction your skin might have when using oils, consult a doctor immediately.

Some essential oils like lemon or orange are sensitive to sunlight—you should only apply those to areas of skin you know won't be exposed to any direct sunlight for at least twelve hours.

Diluted Skin Contact

This is a much gentler way of applying essential oils to your skin. Your body still absorbs the nutrients from the oils, but they aren't as concentrated, and the effects aren't as intense. This method is perfect for those with sensitive skin. Something important to remember is that before you dilute your essential oils with any other products, you have to blend your oils with a carrier oil first.

There are many ways to dilute your essential oils. The most common is to mix them into some of your favorite skincare products, such as lotions, creams, moisturizers, scrubs, etc. Add a few drops of your essential oil blend to your chosen product and mix well. There is no set rule as to how much oil you should use—it works by instinct. You should rarely use more than a few drops, even with larger containers. If you are starting out, you should experiment with smaller amounts first. It's important to write down all your experiments so that you can create your recipes to replicate later. Essential oils work best if you add them to products that are odorless and don't contain any other plant products such as citrus, mint, etc.

Another way to dilute your essential oils is to add them to your bath or shower. There are few things as divine as a relaxing soak with some essential oils to soothe your skin and help you relax. It's easy to add essential oils to your shampoo or liquid soaps. You can also smear a few drops of oil onto your shower wall to inhale the scent while you clean yourself, or you can put some diluted oil onto your washcloth or loofah. If you're taking a bath, you can even pour a few drops right into your bathwater. This not only gives you the benefit of contact with your skin, but you get to enjoy some aromatherapy as well by inhaling the scented steam rising from the water. It's also a good idea to add some essential oils if you make your own bath salts or fizz bombs.

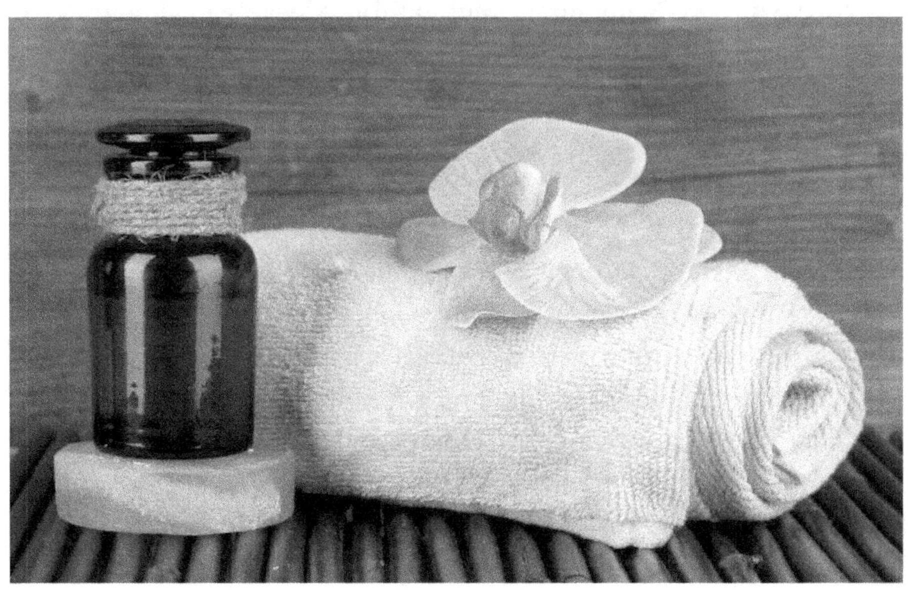

Buying and Storing Essential Oils

The types of oils you buy and where you buy them depend on what you're looking for. When you want essential oil products for aromatherapy, you can buy them from many stores and online retailers. If you want to make your own essential oil creations, or if you are treating a specific condition with the oils, you'll want to purchase therapy-grade oils from a reputable retailer. The more intense the oil grade, the more money you'll spend. Before you buy, consider what you'll be using them for.

Essential oils expire eventually, and it's imperative to store your essential oils properly to obtain as long a lifespan as possible.

Essential oils that have expired can be harmful and should never be used.

There are a few telltale signs that an oil has expired. The first sign is the smell—an expired oil will either lose its scent, or its scent will become stronger and start to smell rancid. The second sign is color. Depending on the type, an expired oil will become lighter, darker, or completely colorless. Expired essential oils can also look cloudy. Lastly, your oil will start to congeal and become thick and lumpy when it expires. Some oils will become so thick that they start to form a paste.

Essential oils generally last a long time—you can keep them for several years if you store them properly. Different types of oils deteriorate at different speeds. Citrus-based oils are the quickest to expire, while wood-based oils tend to improve with time before expiring at a much slower rate. There are, however, a few factors that will increase the rate of deterioration of your oils.

Oxygen

Oxygen is devastating to essential oils, and you should limit exposure as much as possible. The quickest and most effective way is to make sure your oils are kept in airtight containers that are always properly sealed. If you're blending oils, you should close the container immediately after adding the oil. When mixing several oils together, resist the urge to add all the oils first and then put the caps or lids on the bottles, or keep your oils opened during the mixing process in case you need to add more oil. The sooner you close the container, the better. This is also why you shouldn't break the seal of newly-bought oils until the moment you use them for the first time.

Another way to prevent exposure to oxygen is to make sure the container isn't too empty. Less oil inside your container means more space filled with air. If you notice a container is becoming fairly empty, you should transfer the oil into a smaller container or, if you happen to have two bottles of the same essential oil, you can combine the oils so that you have one full container rather than two that are half empty.

Heat and Moisture

Not only does exposure to heat increase the rate of deterioration, but if an essential oil is exposed to intense heat for too long, it may reach temperatures high enough for the oil to combust. Essential oils are highly flammable and should be kept away from open flames and intense heat sources.

Prolonged exposure to moisture is also bad for your oils and will shorten their shelf life. Moisture will eventually turn your oil cloudy, and if too much moisture is caught inside the container, water drops will begin to form, which will dilute your oil and encourage the growth of bacteria. Keeping the cap of your container properly closed will keep moisture from getting inside, but you should keep your oils away from moisture as much as possible.

On their own, heat or moisture can be bad for your oils, but together they will be disastrous. That is why you should never keep your essential oils in the bathroom or the kitchen.

Light

Sunlight is also bad for your oils. The UV radiation in sunlight can cause a chemical reaction that speeds up the rate at which oils expire and weakens the scent and effects of the oils. Essential oils are always sold in dark glass bottles to protect the contents from UV light, but you should still keep your oils out of direct sunlight.

Another problem with sunlight is that it is a source of heat, and prolonged exposure can heat your oil up, which could result in fire. Sudden temperature changes caused by exposing your oils to sunlight and suddenly moving them to somewhere cool will also damage your essential oils.

To summarize, essential oils should always be stored somewhere dark, cool, and dry, and should always be sealed tightly to keep out any air. If you need to transfer your oils into a new container, make sure it is sealable, and stick to glass and stainless steel. Stay away from plastic, as the chemicals in the plastic will react with the oils and ruin them. You also shouldn't leave any oil behind in droppers, as the rubber will react similarly to plastic.

To prolong the shelf life of your oils, you can store them in the fridge, but make sure to keep them separate from your food. Storing essential oils in the fridge is an especially good idea for those who don't use them very often, as frequent users tend to use up all their essential oils before they get a chance to expire.

If the need arises, you can also freeze your essential oils. The oil may become thick and cloudy or even form ice crystals when frozen, but it will return to normal as soon as it reaches room temperature again. You should let the oil defrost naturally—never try to heat it with the oven, microwave, or hairdryer. If you want to speed up the process a little, you can roll the bottle of oil in your hands or place it in a bowl of shallow warm water. When letting your oils defrost, you should always unscrew the cap a little so that it is on loosely. Keep the cap on to protect the oil from exposure to oxygen, but keep it loose to prevent pressure from building inside the bottle as the oil heats up again.

Safety

Essential oils look and smell pretty and come in tiny amounts, but these compounds are extremely powerful. Most commercial products are safe to use and come with specific warnings and instructions. You have to be very careful when applying them.

If you use essential oils on your face or skin, keep them away from your eyes. Always wash your hands thoroughly afterward.

Some final tips on using essential oils safely: remember that they are extremely flammable. Don't burn down your house trying to make it smell nice. Using essential oils during pregnancy is a topic that is currently being debated by consumers, researchers, and healthcare professionals. Use caution and speak to your doctor. You'll also want to keep essential oils out of reach of children.

CHAPTER THREE

How to Blend Essential Oils

Blending is an integral part of using essential oils. Not only will you want to blend different essential oils, but you also need to blend essential oils with carrier oils.

Carrier Oils

Carrier oils are extracted from nuts, seeds, and sometimes bark. They aren't as potent as essential oils and are thus much gentler on the skin. These oils are mainly used to dilute essential oils, making it possible to apply essential oils to the skin without any negative side effects like itching or burning. Most carrier oils have a faint scent, somewhat nutty. This can be an advantage, adding another layer to the scent you've created.

When choosing your carrier oil, you should take into consideration the smell and texture of the carrier oil and the healing properties of each essential oil. Like essential oils, different carrier oils have different properties and should be used for the most suited purposes. All carrier oils should have readily-available information on their labels concerning their healing properties. To help you get started, here are some of the common carrier oils and their uses.

- **Grapeseed oil** is a neutral oil with a faint smell. It is used for almost anything, ranging from skin care to massages to the treatment of sore muscles and bruises. This is a great carrier oil for beginners.
- **Jojoba oil** has a fairly prominent but pleasant smell and is the most commonly used for massage oils. It absorbs easily into the skin, making it ideal for people with oily skin. Its anti-inflammatory properties make it a good option for treating mild cases of acne.

● **Coconut oil** can be used on both the skin and hair and is gentle enough to be applied to the face. Because of its antimicrobial properties, this oil is great for skin care and can be used to protect the skin. It is also one of the few oils that can be used both on its own or as a carrier oil.

● **Olive oil** is common and inexpensive. You can find it in your local grocery store. Just be sure to use "extra virgin" olive oil. This type has more vitamins and minerals than other olive oil.

● **Sweet almond oil** is commonly used because it's rapidly absorbed into your skin and is odorless. It is an excellent skin moisturizer.

● **Rosehip oil** can be used as an antioxidant, and its anti-inflammatory properties make it a great option for treating swelling and various skin conditions. It is also rich in vitamin C and E, making it an excellent choice to help boost your immune system. This oil has a very faint fruity smell.

Another great thing about carrier oils is that you can mix different carrier oils to better personalize the scent and effect you want from your final essential oil blend. The process of blending essential oils into carrier oils is simple. In a sealable container—preferably stainless steel or glass—measure out your carrier oil or oils and add a few drops of your favorite essential oil or oil blend. You can either stir the mixture or seal the container and give it a good shake. Your diluted oil mixture is ready to be used and should be stored the same way undiluted essential oils are stored.

There are no set rules on the exact dilution ratio between essential oils and carrier oils, and directions vary from source to source, but there are a few guidelines:

● If diluting oils with the intent of using them on children, you should limit the essential oils to a ratio of 1%, meaning no more than 6 drops of essential oil per full oz of carrier oil.

● For fully grown, healthy adults, the general ratio is 2.5%, or 15 drops per oz. The standard ratio for a proper aromatherapy session is 3 percent (20 drops per oz).

● To treat targeted problems like muscle pain, headaches, acne, etc., you can use a ratio of 5 to 10%, meaning 30 to 60 drops per oz. With these higher dilution ratios, you should be very careful and test the mixture on your skin for itching or burning before applying to the affected area.

Like essential oils, carrier oils should be tested for allergic reactions, and you should not use an expired carrier oil.

Mixing Essential Oils

Combining essential oils to create new scents can be a fun and relaxing hobby. Even as a beginner, you can never go wrong if you're happy with your final result. However, creating interesting new scents is still an art form that takes skill, knowledge, and practice. There are nuances and layers to developing scents that are often overlooked and underappreciated.

The first thing you need to understand when making complex scents is that there are different *notes* in every scent. Notes are all the different aromas within the scent and can be classified into three basic types: *top note, middle note,* and *base note.* The top note is the first aroma you notice in a scent. It is prominent and sharp and usually doesn't last very long. This note usually creates the main characteristics of the scent. The middle note is a slightly subtler aroma that lasts a little longer than the top note and forms the heart of the scent. When applied to a sample strip, it should last roughly an hour or two. The base note is a scent that isn't immediately noticeable and starts to become more prominent a little later. In some cases, a base note can take a few hours or even a whole day before it becomes prominent on a perfume strip and will last a fairly long time. The base note is incredibly important, as it determines how long your scent will last. The stronger your base note, the stronger your final scent.

There are discrepancies about which essential oils fall into which note type. With some research or experimentation, it will be easy to categorize the oils yourself. Figuring out your notes is part of the whole scent mixing process. Here are some basic steps to guide you.

1. To get started, choose a few essential oils you like. This may seem a little difficult if you start overthinking it, but this is a fairly easy step that can be instinctive. Ask yourself which flowers you like to smell, what are your favorite herbs and spices, and which fruit calls to you. You can also complete this step by smelling testers of different oils and choosing the ones you like the most.

2. Once you have all the oils you like, cut a piece of paper to make perfume strips for each one. Put a drop of each oil onto its perfume strip and label the strips.

3. Start testing each oil by gradually bringing the perfume strip closer to your nose. You may also want to draw circles with the strip and alternate between deep and shallow breaths. Take note of how close the strip is before smelling it to see how strong each scent is.

4. As you test the strip, try to find words that describe the properties of the smell of the oil. These words can be anything, from shapes and textures—like sharp, smooth, rough, grainy, rounded—to personality traits—like aggressive, friendly, gentle, etc.—to sounds and colors they bring to mind or memories you associate with the different smell. You can also use descriptive words like fruity, woody, sensual, sweet, loud, heavy, etc. Once again, don't overthink this and try to analyze the scent scientifically. Simply write down whatever comes to mind as you breathe in the smell of the oil. If you need to close your eyes to help visualize, go right ahead.

5. Once you've tested each of the perfume strips and taken notes, let the samples rest for roughly half an hour. Use this opportunity to breathe in some fresh air or smell some coffee beans to refresh your sense of smell.

6. Once the samples have rested, repeat the test in steps 3 and 4. Make notes on how each scent has changed. Some may have faded or become stronger. Some undertones, descriptive words, and associated colors may have shifted slightly. You can let the samples rest again, redo the test, and take notes at intervals throughout the day. There is no rush when mixing a new scent, and you should always take your time during these tests.

7. From your notes and observations, you should be able to categorize the different oils into top notes, middle notes, and base notes. Once you've done that, it's time to choose the oils you want to use. Use your notes to help you find the oils that you think will work well together and complement each other. If you're planning on using a blend for specific healing purposes, you should take the healing properties of each oil—which should be listed on the label of the oil—into consideration. As a starting point, choose five oils. Once you've had some practice mixing basic new scents, you can move on to experimenting with larger combinations. Ideally, you should have two top notes, two middle notes, and one base note.

8. Next, you need to figure out the ratio of the different oils. Even though you can calculate the ratio by using the strength of each scent, the best way to find the balance that works for you is through experimentation. You'll need several wooden skewers, cotton buds, or perfume strips for this. Put a drop of each oil on several pieces of your chosen medium. I will be using cotton buds as an example for this phase.

9. Mix and match your oil samples until you have a combination you think might work, e.g., three parts oil one, eight parts oil two, two parts oil three, five parts oil four, and six parts oil five. Use one cotton bud for each part. Create a fan with your selected cotton buds and waft them in front of your nose. Take deep breaths of the combined scent to determine how you feel about it. It may not be perfect yet, and some oils may be too strong or too weak. If an oil is coming on too strongly, remove one or two cotton buds. If an oil isn't strong enough, add a few cotton buds. Keep playing

around with your combinations until you find the perfect balance for the scent you're creating. Keep thorough notes on what you're doing.

10.	Before settling on a final recipe, place your chosen combination of oil samples in a sealed container and let it rest for 30 minutes to an hour. Then, open the container and breathe in the scent. The scent will likely have changed slightly and developed new depths and layers. Make a few final adjustments to your combination and write down the recipe. You may want to convert your recipe to percentages. To do this, divide the number of the parts of each oil by the total number of parts, then multiply that by 100. That should give you the percentage of each oil.

11.	Now that you've created your recipe, mix larger amounts of oil in a suitable container to create your new blend. This blend is ready to be used immediately or stored for later. Make sure you label your blend correctly and keep all of your notes, not just the recipe, somewhere safe and organized.

You can repeat this process as many times as you want to create new blends. When blending for specific healing purposes, the process may become a little more difficult, and you may not always know where to start. To help you with that, the last few chapters of this book will offer effective aromatherapy recipes for skin care, hair care, pain relief, stress relief, allergies, and other common ailments.

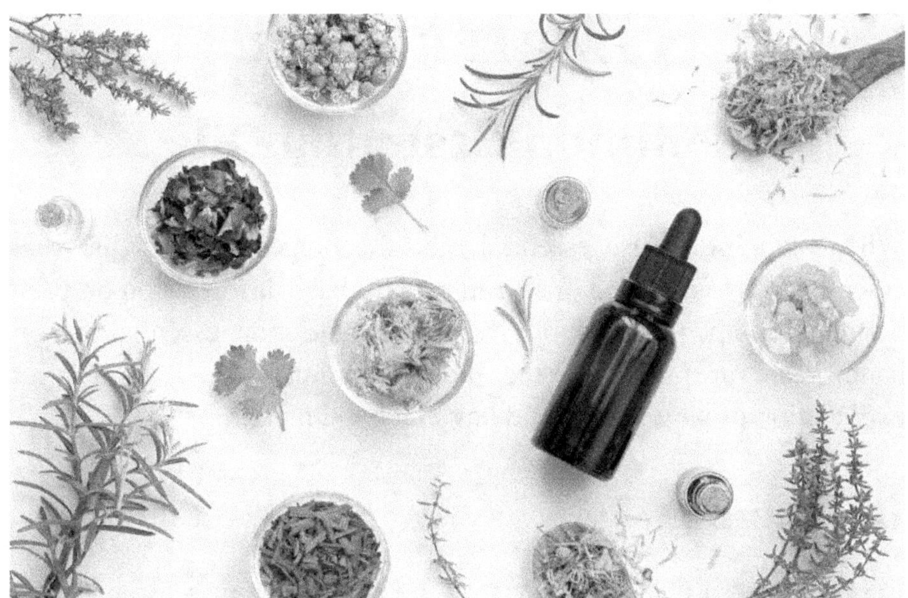

CHAPTER FOUR

Common Essential Oils

When planning to use essential oils, the biggest question is what essential oils to buy first. You can usually base this decision on each particular recipe you find, but it's best to have some essential oils on hand. Here are some of the most common ones, with a brief explanation of why you should have them on hand.

Bergamot

Bergamot has a pleasing scent that can enhance your sense of peace and happiness, and it's a popular oil for room diffusers. Use it as an antiseptic, an antidepressant, and even as a deodorant, but be careful about using it undiluted on the skin, as it can irritate sensitive skin. Blend it into your bath if you're feeling anxious or fearful. Bergamot also happens to be one of the main ingredients of Earl Grey tea.

Cinnamon

Cinnamon is an herb that originated in central Asia and is widely used in healing treatments throughout India and Sri Lanka. It's good for more than flavoring your cider and giving your holiday decorations a burst of seasonal scents. It boosts brain function, increases blood circulation, and helps your body fight off infection. Use cinnamon oil to repel mosquitoes as well. Studies have shown that it's effective in killing larvae.

Chamomile

Chamomile is another relaxant and mood booster that will do wonders for your mental health and general state of mind, especially when combined with lavender or rose. Chamomile tea is one of the most widely-used ways to relieve stress and help wind down after a hard or emotional day.

Clove

Clove essential oil is full of antioxidants and has pain-relieving properties. It is also widely used in dental work. Clove oil has antibacterial, antifungal, and antiseptic characteristics. When used in a diffuser, it helps kill airborne microorganisms. When diluted, it can treat cuts, scrapes, and bites.

Eucalyptus

One of the most common essential oils used by nearly everyone is eucalyptus. You might have been using it for years without realizing it. This oil is found in many household, health, and beauty products because it's a powerful agent for clearing up respiratory illnesses. It can calm a cough, make your scratchy throat feel better, and help eliminate lung congestion. Keep in mind that this essential oil is highly potent, so keep it away from your eyes.

Frankincense

Frankincense essential oil is known to be great for your skin, and it's also considered to have spiritual properties, with many mental and emotional benefits when used correctly. It is used in many topical recipes as well as in a diffuser.

Grapefruit

Some of the most common essential oils come from citrus fruits, which are packed with vitamins, minerals, and antioxidants that help you fight diseases. Grapefruit oil is created by cold pressing the fruit's rind to extract its essence. It has been useful as an antidepressant. Use it in a diffuser or dilute it and spray on your linens.

Geranium

From the leaves of what might be a favorite flower, geranium essential oil is useful due to its citronellol and geraniol. These compounds influence your brain and nervous system, helping you control your emotions and resist the temptation to become angry or irritable. *When ingested, this type of oil may have toxic effects, so use it as an inhalant or an aromatic.*

Jasmine

Jasmine oil is an excellent antidepressant and a muscle relaxant that can make childbirth easier and soothe cramps and pain. It can also be used to boost libido.

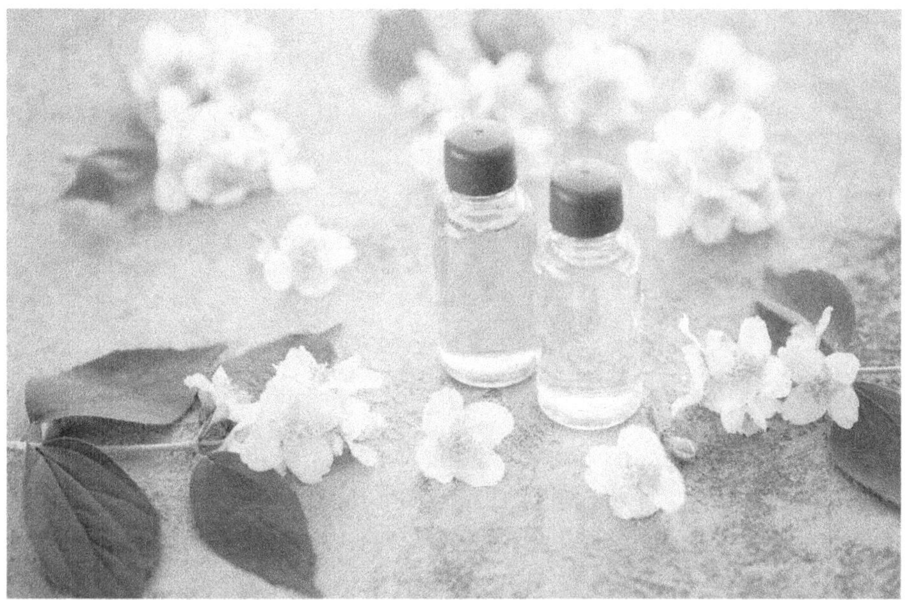

Lavender

Lavender oil is probably the most commonly used essential oil out there. It is often used simply for its lovely floral smell, but it is great for relieving stress and relaxing the mind. For help with sleeping, drop a bit of lavender oil on your pillow.

Lemon

Lemon is another popular oil that is used for its scent. It is also suitable for treating headaches, aiding digestion, and boosting your mood. Because of its strong acidity, it is ideal for adding to cleaning supplies to help burn through grime and dirt and get rid of bacteria. It is also rich in vitamin C, which helps fight illnesses and can help treat colds.

Mint

Mint is a scent that's often associated with freshness and certain types of candy and is used frequently in all its forms, including as an essential oil. Not only does mint bring with it a breath of fresh air, but it is excellent for aiding digestion and giving your mind and body an extra boost of energy.

Oregano

Oregano oil is high in phenol, which means it's highly effective in cleansing receptor spots of the body. It's most commonly used in the Raindrop Technique for healing. In this process, several drops of oregano essential oil are put on the spine and massaged into the back, which is good for muscle tension and pain and strengthens your immune system. It contains a number of antioxidant properties. Physically, it will open up your respiratory system and help you breathe. Mentally, it can induce feelings of safety and security.

Peppermint

Peppermint essential oil contains a lot of nutrients and minerals, such as vitamin C and potassium. It's one of the oldest essential oils used today, and the relative ease with which the oil can be extracted from peppermint leaves and bark makes it abundant. Put peppermint oil into your bathwater to enjoy the aromatherapy and relax your nerves.

Rose

Rose is another essential oil often used purely for its scent. It also works great for reducing anxiety and boosting your overall mood. This makes it a good option for aromatherapy and creating a calm, relaxed atmosphere around the house.

Rosemary

Rosemary is a Mediterranean herb that's popular with Italian and Greek cooking. Rosemary oil has more to offer than culinary delights. It's excellent for hair care, stimulating follicle growth, and can be used with shampoo. It also positively affects your mood and provides a burst of energy. Try inhaling it when you're studying, trying to focus on a project, or need an adrenaline jolt.

Sandalwood

Sandalwood is a strong, aromatic oil that works well for focusing the mind and calming your nerves. A combination of sandalwood and mint can be a great way to help you get through a long, stressful day at work.

Sweet Orange

This essential oil can be used in your bath, degreaser, or lotion. It is even a great oil to diffuse to help you stay focused but relaxed.

Tea Tree

Tea Tree can be used as an immune booster and to ward off infections and illnesses. It can help treat skin conditions and is a powerful antimicrobial.

Ylang-Ylang

Ylang-Ylang is great for the skin and is often used to treat troublesome skin conditions. It can also be used to soothe headaches and ease nausea.

These are just some of the most common essential oils used worldwide. When you buy them, be sure to follow any specific instructions. Remember that they are very powerful and heavily concentrated, so a little goes a long way. If you're working with oil you've never used before, it's best to start with a small quantity and slowly add to it if you feel you need more.

CHAPTER FIVE

Essential Oil Blends for Skin Care

Skin care is a popular reason to use essential oils. People have successfully treated chronic skin conditions, healed wounds, and improved the look and feel of their skin with essential oils. You'll also find body scrubs and moisturizers in this chapter to suit your beauty needs.

Stretch Mark Reducing Blend

Stretch marks can make people feel uncomfortable with their bodies, but you can reduce the visibility of stretch marks with this recipe.

Ingredients:
5 drops Frankincense Oil
5 drops Myrrh Oil
5 drops Grapefruit Oil
¼ cup Coconut Oil

Directions:
1. Melt your coconut oil before mixing it with essential oils.
2. Let it cool, and apply to stretch marks up to three times daily.

Scar Salve

No one wants to deal with unsightly scars, but you can seldom get rid of scars completely. With this scar salve, however, you can reduce noticeable scars over time.

Ingredients:
20 drops Frankincense Oil

20 drops Helichrysum Oil

20 drops Lavender Oil

1 oz. Beeswax

2 oz. Shea Butter

3 oz. Coconut Oil

Directions:

1. Melt your coconut oil and shea butter over medium heat.

2. Add the beeswax, and stir gently until the wax is melted completely. Let it cool for five minutes.

3. Stir in the essential oils.

4. Store in an airtight container. Close your container once the mixture is cool. A 5-oz. container is suggested, as this recipe makes five ounces.

5. Apply two to three times each day.

Whipped Eczema Cream

Eczema is a painful skin condition that spreads if it isn't taken care of. This eczema cream is potent and soothing, making it easy to use.

Ingredients:

¼ cup Shea Butter

¼ cup Coconut Oil

15 drops Lavender Oil

5–6 drops Tea Tree Oil

Directions:

1. Using a double boiler, melt your shea butter and coconut oil.

2. Remove from the heat and let cool for up to five minutes.

3. Gently add the essential oils before scooping the mixture into a bowl.

4. Beat on high until whipped, and spoon into a glass jar.

5. Rub onto affected areas twice a day.

Whipped Body Butter

Moisturizing your skin is important for its health. If you have moisturized skin properly, it'll appear softer and even brighter.

Ingredients:

1¾ cup Unrefined Shea Butter

½ cup Extra Virgin Coconut Oil

¼ cup Grapeseed Oil

20 drops Sweet Orange Oil

15 drops Lemon Oil

Directions:

1. Add your coconut oil and unrefined shea butter to a double boiler. You'll need to melt it slowly, stirring constantly so that there are no lumps.

2. Let cool slightly before adding grapeseed oil and essential oils.

3. Let cool until solid again, and then whip on high.

4. Put into a glass jar and apply to skin to moisturize it and relax tense muscles.

Wrinkle Cream

You don't have to be old to get wrinkles. Different people will get wrinkles at different times, but you can benefit from this wrinkle-reduction cream no matter your age.

Ingredients:

¼ cup Shea Butter

¼ cup Organic Coconut Oil

7–10 drops Lavender Oil

10–12 drops Frankincense Oil

Directions:

1. Melt your coconut oil and shea butter. It's best to use a double boiler and then let it cool.

2. Make sure you gently add the essential oils, mixing thoroughly.

3. Let the mixture cool to room temperature, and apply each night before bed to reduce wrinkles. It should be applied after cleaning your face and patting it dry.

Natural Toner

Everyone can benefit from a toner to eliminate excess toxins and oils, but not everyone has the money to spend on this treatment. This essential oil toner, however, is cheap and easy to make.

Ingredients:

8 oz. Water

2 drops Lavender Oil

2 drops Geranium Oil

2 drops Frankincense Oil

Directions:

1. Mix together and put into a bottle.

2. Shake well before using, and dip a cotton ball into it to apply gently to your skin. Only apply after washing and patting your face dry.

Oil Blend for Age Spots

No matter your age, you'll find that you have some sort of blemish. These blemishes can turn into age spots as you get older, and no one wants to deal with that. Using this one essential oil correctly, you can reduce your age spots in no time.

Ingredients:

6 drops Frankincense Oil

½ teaspoon Vitamin E Oil

Directions:

1. Mix and apply directly to your skin.

Sweet Sugar Scrub

This sugar scrub is meant to exfoliate the skin, making it softer and brighter. You should not allow dead skin cells to pile up and make your skin look bad and feel even worse.

Ingredients:

2 cups White Sugar

½ cup Coconut Oil, melted

7–10 drops Orange Oil

3–5 drops Vanilla Extract

Directions:

1. Combine the sugar and coconut oil in a bowl.

2. Add the orange oil and vanilla extract. Stir to mix well.

3. Store the mixture in a widemouthed container with a tight lid.

4. Scrub the blend over the skin to exfoliate and cleanse, keeping away from the eyes.

5. Rinse away with warm water and pat dry.

Bath Bomb for Skin Care

Ingredients:

2 cups Baking Soda

1 cup Sea Salt

1 cup Citric Acid

1 cup Corn Starch

1 tablespoon Jojoba Oil
30 drops Tea Tree Oil
30 drops Lemon Oil
20 drops Lavender Oil
60 ml Witch Hazel in a Spray Bottle

Directions:

1. Mix all the ingredients except the witch hazel in a container.

2. While mixing, moisten the mixture with the witch hazel spray.

3. Pack the mixture into ice cube molds, and let them dry overnight.

4. Take the bath bombs out of the molds and air-dry for two more days before using them in your bath.

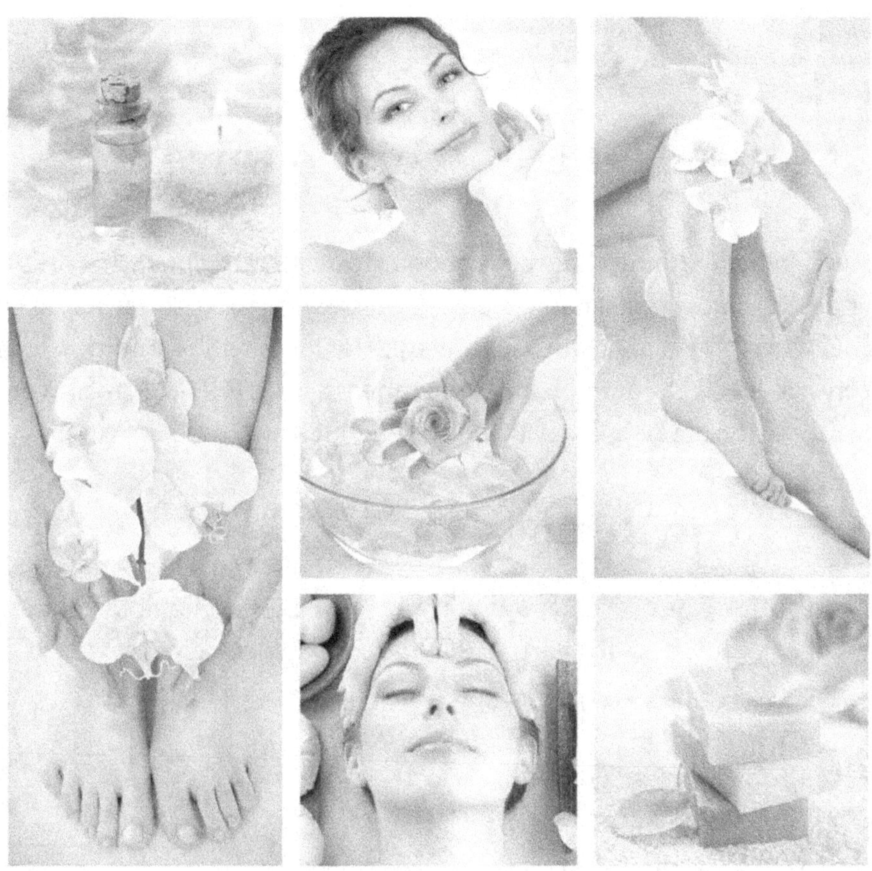

CHAPTER SIX

Essential Oil Recipes for Acne

Acne isn't something that most people want to talk about, but it is a condition that affects most teens. You do not need to suffer from acne when you can use essential oils to lessen the condition and even get rid of it completely. Remember that different recipes work best for different people. If you have bad luck with one, try another.

Easy Acne Recipe

If you suffer from acne, you don't want to have a ridiculous amount of upkeep. It's best to start with this easy acne recipe to see if it works.

Ingredients:
6 drops Frankincense Oil
4 drops Lavender Oil
2 drops Tea Tree Oil
30 ml of Jojoba Oil

Directions:
1. Mix your essential oils with the jojoba oil. Apply to areas that are acne-prone right before bed every night.

Blackheads Begone

Many people consider blackheads as bad as regular pimples, but there's no reason to fear. This simple baking soda and lemon oil recipe will take care of them in one treatment.
Ingredients:

1 teaspoon Baking Soda
1 teaspoon Water
2–3 drops Lemon Oil

Directions:
1. Mix together until a paste is formed, and apply to the area.
2. Leave it on for twenty to twenty-five minutes before washing off gently.
3. Pat your skin dry.

Pimple Pop Roller

If you don't want to make an acne-fighting recipe every time you need it, just get a roller bottle for this wonderful acne recipe.

Ingredients:
15 drops Tea Tree Oil
15 drops Lavender Oil
15 drops Frankincense Oil
Carrier Oil (Sweet Almond Oil Suggested)

Directions:
1. Combine in a roller bottle, topping the mixture with a carrier oil. A 10-ml roller bottle is suggested.
2. Apply to affected areas or areas of concern before bed each night.

Acne Treatment Cream

Some people are hesitant to put more oil on their acne-prone skin, but this acne-fighting cream will help.

Ingredients:
¼ cup Coconut Oil

10 drops Tea Tree Oil

10 drops Lemon Oil

10 drops Lavender Oil

Directions:

1. Melt your coconut oil and add the essential oils.

2. Make sure that you don't use a metal spoon. The metal will react with these oils and weaken the strength of your mixture.

3. Put into the refrigerator until firm.

4. Dab on affected areas in the morning and evening after you clean and dry your face.

Herbal Face Scrub for Acne

Ingredients:

250 ml Oatmeal, finely ground

125 ml Carrier Oil (Sweet Almond Oil Suggested)

1 tablespoon Dry Herbs (Lemongrass, Witch Hazel, Lavender Flowers, or Rose Flower Petals), finely ground

1 teaspoon Spices (Cinnamon Powder or Turmeric Powder)

30 drops Tea Tree Oil

30 drops Lemon Oil

20 drops Lavender Oil

Directions:

1. Mix the ingredients in a widemouthed container with a tight lid.

2. Rub the blend onto your face, but keep away from the eyes. After some time, rinse off with lukewarm water.

Tip: Never scrub your face if you have any swollen acne lacerations.

CHAPTER SEVEN

Essential Oil Blends for Hair Care

From helping an itchy scalp, getting rid of dandruff, and renewing hair growth to ridding yourself of lice naturally, essential oils can help. With these wonderful recipes, you can take care of your hair in no time.

Itchy Scalp Remedy

An itchy scalp can strike at any time, but most people don't realize that an itchy scalp means an unhealthy scalp. Use this essential oil mixture to heal your scalp.

Ingredients:
15 drops Lavender Oil
15 drops Lemon Oil
10 drops Tea Tree Oil
1½ cups Water
½ cup Witch Hazel

Directions:
1. Mix everything in a spray bottle, and mist your hair after washing or before brushing. You can do this two to three times daily.

Anti-Dandruff Shampoo

A variety of things can cause dandruff, but no matter the cause, this anti-dandruff recipe can help. With lavender essential oil, you'll even get a soothing effect after a long, stressful day.
Ingredients:

5 drops Tea Tree Oil
2 drops Lavender Oil
1 drop Rosemary Oil
2 drops Copaiba Oil

Directions:

1. Add the essential oils to your shampoo treatment for that day (not the bottle).

2. Apply directly to your scalp, and let it sit for one to two minutes before washing.

Dry Scalp Cure

A dry scalp can be itchy, but it can also just be a pain all on its own. This recipe is easy to make and easy to use. You can even mix it into your conditioner.

Ingredients:

6 drops Cedarwood Oil
2 drops Patchouli Oil
2 drops Geranium Oil
1 teaspoon Coconut Oil

Directions:

1. Mix everything together, and massage gently into your dry scalp.

2. Cover with a towel for a minimum of fifteen minutes, and then shampoo and thoroughly rinse your hair twice.

Deep Hair Conditioner

You don't need to pay salon prices to get a deep conditioning treatment that works without the chemicals. You'll find that this all-natural, essential oil-infused recipe does wonders for the health and shine of your hair.

Ingredients:

15 drops Rosewood Oil

9 drops Sandalwood Oil

9 drops Lavender Oil

½ cup Olive Oil

Directions:

1. Mix everything in a bag, and warm up gently in warm water by dunking the bag into it.

2. Apply it to your hair, wrapping your hair for twenty to twenty-five minutes.

3. Shampoo and wash your hair as usual.

Hair Moisturizer

Ingredients:

1 oz. Jojoba Oil (if you have black hair, use Camellia Oil)

12 drops Cedarwood Oil

12 drops Lavender Oil

8 drops Rosemary Oil

Directions:

1. Combine all the ingredients in a PET plastic bottle.

2. After mixing them well, massage about a teaspoonful of the combination into your hair and scalp.

3. Use a shower cap and wrap your hair using a warm, moistened towel. Wait for a minimum of fifteen minutes, and then shampoo and thoroughly rinse your hair twice.

4. Dry it and then style it as you usually do. This can be done weekly or monthly.

Beard Oil Recipe

If you have a beard or just want to give the gift of all-natural beard oil, this recipe is great. Beard hair can be hard to tame, but this recipe will make it smoother and more manageable.

Ingredients:
½ oz. Argon Oil
¼ oz. Sweet Almond Oil
¼ oz. Jojoba Oil
7 drops Lavender Oil
5 drops Rosemary Oil
3 drops Cedarwood Oil

Directions:
1. Mix together and put into a glass bottle with a dropper.
2. Drop three to five drops into your hand, and work through your beard. If you have a longer beard, you may need more drops, but add a small amount at a time so that you do not oversaturate the hair.

DIY Lice Treatment

Unfortunately, lice affect many people no matter how hard they try to avoid them, but you don't need to rely on chemical-laced shampoos if you use this essential oil treatment.

Ingredients:
1 cup Olive Oil
20 drops Tea Tree Oil
20 drops Lavender Oil

Directions:
1. Mix together and apply to your hair.
2. Leave the mixture on for an hour before combing your hair.

3. Shampoo twice to rinse the mixture thoroughly.

CHAPTER EIGHT

Essential Oil Blends for Stress Relief

Stress is an inevitable part of life, but there are a number of essential oils that can help relieve feelings of anxiety or panic. There are also many different ways in which you can apply these oils.

Soothing Blend for Anxiety

There's no shame in having anxiety, but you shouldn't sit back and do nothing. To get rid of anxiety naturally, you'll find that this simple blend helps immensely.

Ingredients:
10 drops Lavender Oil
4 drops Rosemary Oil

Directions:
1. Diffuse the oils in a diffuser to reduce stress.

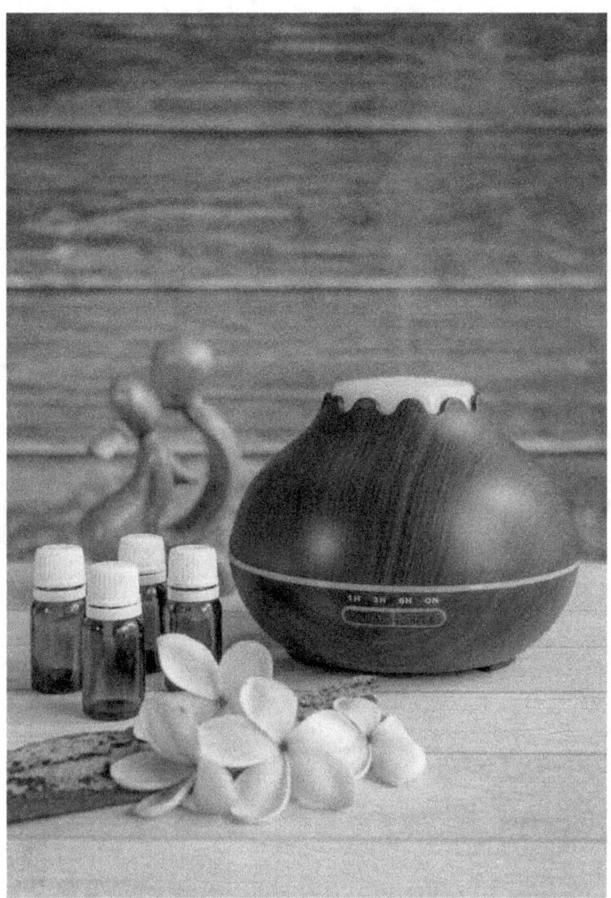

Relaxing Blend for Stress Relief

Ingredients:
30 drops Cedarwood Oil
30 drops Ylang Ylang Oil
25 drops Lavender Oil
20 drops Patchouli Oil
20 drops Bergamot Oil
Jojoba Oil (optional)

Directions:

1. Mix all the essential oils in a dark glass vial. Dilute the mixture with the jojoba oil if desired.

2. Take a few drops, rub them between your palms, and deeply inhale the scent for an immediate calming effect when you are in anxious or stressful situations.

3. You can add a few drops to warm bathwater for a peaceful and tranquilizing bath.

Stress Relieving Bath

You should use this mixture once a week and make sure that you soak for at least twenty minutes. It'll help lower your stress-related hormones, balance your pH level, and even pull out toxins.

Ingredients:
½ cup Epsom Salt
10 drops Lavender Oil
½ cup Baking Soda
4 drops Rose Oil
Directions:
1. Mix the ingredients, and put them into warm bathwater.

2. Soak for twenty minutes, and then continue your bath like normal.

Lavender Remedy for Insomnia

Insomnia is a big source of stress. You can't do much about it besides trying to relax, but one essential oil can help you relax to kick insomnia out of your life.

Ingredients:
Lavender Oil

Directions:

1. Just put a few drops of lavender oil on your pillow, and you'll rest a little easier.

2. Reapply once a week.

Sleepy Time Bath

Maybe it hasn't gotten as far as insomnia, but you'll find that poor sleep creates a bad mood. This bath is designed to help you relax enough to get a good night's rest right afterward.

Ingredients:
10 drops Lavender Oil
7 drops Roman Chamomile Oil
¼ cup Sea Salt
1 tablespoon Jojoba Oil
Directions:
1. Mix everything together, and then add to a warm bath. Soak for about twenty minutes.

Quick Relaxation

Relaxing is a great way to improve your mood because tension will make for a bad day and even a severe headache. You'll notice the effects of this blend in as little as five minutes.

Ingredients:
½ teaspoon Sweet Almond Oil
2–4 drops Chamomile Oil
4 drops Lavender Oil
3 drops Peppermint Oil

Directions:
1. Mix together and apply directly to your temples.

Calm a Child

Children can be hard to calm down, and they have bad days just like adults. This essential oil blend is great to keep on hand, and you can use it in advance to keep your children calm and happy.

Ingredients:
25 drops Chamomile Oil
25 drops Lavender Oil
½ cup Water

Directions:
1. Put into a spritzer bottle and spray on stuffed animals or bedding to help calm upset children.

CHAPTER NINE

Essential Oil Blends for Pain Relief

Pain comes in many different forms, from arthritis to migraines to muscle pain. People deal with pain throughout their lives, but you do not have to put up with it. These simple essential oil recipes can be used to soothe pain.

Quick Relief Blend for Arthritis

No one should have to deal with joint pain, and you don't have to just deal with your arthritis. This simple blend is easy to make and provides quick relief.

Ingredients:
5 drops Peppermint Oil
4 drops Chamomile Oil
4 drops Eucalyptus Oil
30 ml Carrier Oil (Sweet Almond Oil Suggested)

Directions:
1. Mix together and rub into joints as needed. You'll need to create this mixture each time.

Migraine Remedy

Migraines in different forms plague many people, and all you need for this migraine relief blend is a roller bottle. You should notice relief in just fifteen minutes.

Ingredients:
5 drops Peppermint Oil
5 drops Lavender Oil

Carrier Oil (Sunflower Oil Suggested)

5 drops Rosemary Oil

Directions:

1. Mix all your essential oils in a roller vial.

2. Add your carrier oil until the vial is full. Shake well.

3. Take a few drops on your fingers and gently massage your forehead, temples, and back of your neck. Keep away from the eyes. Always shake well before using.

Aromatherapy Bath for Migraines

This bath recipe is for a migraine or headache due to hormonal problems or lack of sleep. When used for the proper migraine, it should help immensely.

Ingredients:

5 drops Sandalwood Oil

2 tablespoons Baking Soda

1 tablespoon Jojoba Oil

10 drops Chamomile Oil

10 drops Peppermint Oil

Directions:

1. Mix all ingredients, and then put into warm bathwater. Soak for about thirty minutes or more.

Muscle Relaxer

This muscle rub is easy to make and even easier to put on once it's been in a roller bottle. It has a cool, soothing effect, so you'll feel better in as little as ten minutes.

Ingredients:

5 drops Peppermint Oil

3 drops Clove Oil
5 drops Wintergreen Oil
3 drops Black Pepper Oil
Carrier Oil (Vitamin E Suggested)

Directions:

1. Mix all essential oils in the roller bottle, and then top off with carrier oil.

2. Shake well each time before using. Gently rub the blend into sore areas.

Soothing Bath for Muscle Tension

Muscle tension doesn't always need a cream. You'll find that this bath can help just as much, and it's a lot easier to use when you don't feel like doing anything but soaking your troubles away.

Ingredients:

10 drops Lavender Oil
5 drops Peppermint Oil
5 drops Citrus Oil
3 drops Clove Oil
1 tablespoon Jojoba Oil

Directions:

1. Mix all the ingredients before adding to your bathwater, and then soak for at least thirty minutes.

Basic Pain Relief Salve

This is an all-around pain relief salve. It does take about thirty minutes to make, but you'll find you can use it many times. It even keeps up to six to eight months.

Ingredients:

40 drops Eucalyptus Oil

10 drops Rosemary Oil

20 drops Clove Oil

40 drops Peppermint Oil

¼ cup Coconut Oil

¾ cup Sunflower Oil

1 teaspoon Vitamin E Oil

4 tablespoons Beeswax granules

¼ teaspoon Cayenne Pepper

Directions:

1. Use a double boiler, and combine the sunflower oil with coconut oil. Then add the beeswax over medium heat. Make sure to stir gently until melted.

2. Add your cayenne pepper and stir. Let it cool for five minutes.

3. Add your essential oils and vitamin E oil. Make sure you mix slowly and gently.

4. Pour the mixture into a glass container. Let it cool until the liquid turns into a solid.

5. Store at room temperature.

6. When you want to use it, scoop a small amount, and massage into the painful area.

CHAPTER TEN

Essential Oil Recipes for Allergies and Sunburn

There is so much more that you can do with essential oils. You can use them to help relieve allergies and heal a sunburn.

Allergy Relief

Allergies can affect you at the worst times and even cause problems throughout the year for certain individuals. Not everyone wants to take allergy medicine or even has it on hand, but certain essential oils can relieve the worst of the symptoms.

Ingredients:
¼ teaspoon Sweet Almond Oil
2 drops Lavender Oil
3 drops Frankincense Oil

Directions:
1. Mix together and rub on your palms before inhaling deeply. This should help relieve allergy symptoms, such as itchy eyes and throat irritation.

Allergy Relief Bath

With this wonderful bath, you'll find that your allergies wouldn't bother you. It's a great way to start or end your day to get the relief you need during the worst days of any allergy season.

Ingredients:
¼ cup Epsom Salt

1 tablespoon Sesame Seed Oil

5 drops Basil Oil

10 drops Lavender Oil

Directions:

1. Combine all ingredients before adding to warm bathwater.

2. Soak for at least twenty minutes.

Poison Ivy Treatment

Poison ivy is difficult to deal with, but you'll find relief with this blend, which is also effective for treating poison oak.

Ingredients:

3 drops Peppermint Oil

½ teaspoon Coconut Oil

Directions:

1. Melt the coconut oil, and mix in the essential oil.

2. Using a cotton ball, apply the blend to the affected area three times a day.

Essential Oil Remedy for Sunburn

Sunburn can happen at any time of the year, and severity will always vary. This essential oil blend will help provide quick, soothing relief.

Ingredients:

1 tablespoon Coconut Oil

7 drops Lavender Oil

7 drops Chamomile Oil

Directions:

1. Melt your coconut oil, and mix in the essential oils.

2. When cooled down, apply to your sunburn with a cotton ball. This should help reduce the swelling and pain.

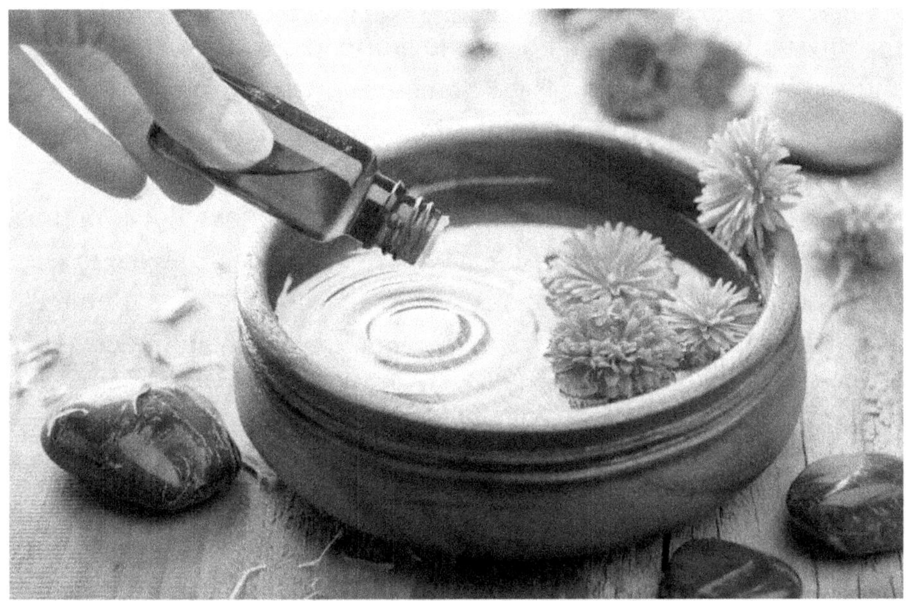

CHAPTER ELEVEN

Essential Oil Blends for the Home

Essential oils can be used around the house to create beautiful scents and for more specific purposes. Sometimes, when mixing your own blends, you'll end up with something you aren't necessarily happy with. Rather than throwing these experiments away, you can add these to your water when washing the floors or windows or mix them with your wood polish. This way, you can spread lovely, subtle scents throughout the house. In many cases, the oils used have antiseptic or antimicrobial properties that actually help the cleaning process.

Here are some recipes for essential oil blends that will be useful around the house.

Air Freshener Blend

Ingredients:
5 drops Wild Orange Oil
5 drops Lemon Oil
5 drops Grapefruit Oil

Directions:
1. Mix the essential oils in a dark glass vial.
2. Use this blend in a diffuser, humidifier, or diluted in a spray bottle as an air freshener.

Disinfectant Blend

This blend works great as a disinfectant that you can use to clean your hands, tiles, counters, basins, toilets, floors, etc.

Ingredients:
5 drops Lavender Oil
5 drops Tea Tree Oil
2 drops Wild Orange Oil

Directions:
1. Mix the essential oils in a dark glass vial.
2. Simply dilute the blend in a spray bottle with distilled water and use it as a disinfectant.

Cleaning Scrub

Here is a recipe for a scrub for cleaning sinks, bathtubs, and tiles.

Ingredients:
10 drops Lemon Oil
10 drops Wild Orange Oil
10 drops Peppermint Oil
1 cup Baking Soda
Water

Directions:
1. In a bowl, combine the baking soda, essential oils, and 3 tablespoons water.
2. Add more water (2–3 tablespoons) to make a liquid paste. Mix well.
3. Store the mixture in a widemouthed container with a tight lid.

Natural Pest Repellent

Use this blend both inside and outside the house as a natural pest repellent. It's safe for all your plants and can be used safely around children and pets.

Ingredients:
14 drops Lavender Oil
7 drops Sweet Orange Oil
7 drops Mint Oil
7 drops Cedarwood Oil
1 cup water

Directions:
1. In a dark spray bottle, mix the essential oils with water.
2. Use as a pest repellent spray.

Conclusion

Essential oils can be used for many different purposes. Whether you are new to essential oils and just learning how to use them, have an interest in making your own essential oils, or dream of making your perfumes using these fabulous tools, I hope this book has managed to help you along your journey. Use the knowledge in this book to improve the quality of your life and the lives of your loved ones. Feel free to share your knowledge with others and spread the love of essential oils. I hope you enjoy the results of reading this book and have tons of fun experimenting with oils and creating your new blends.

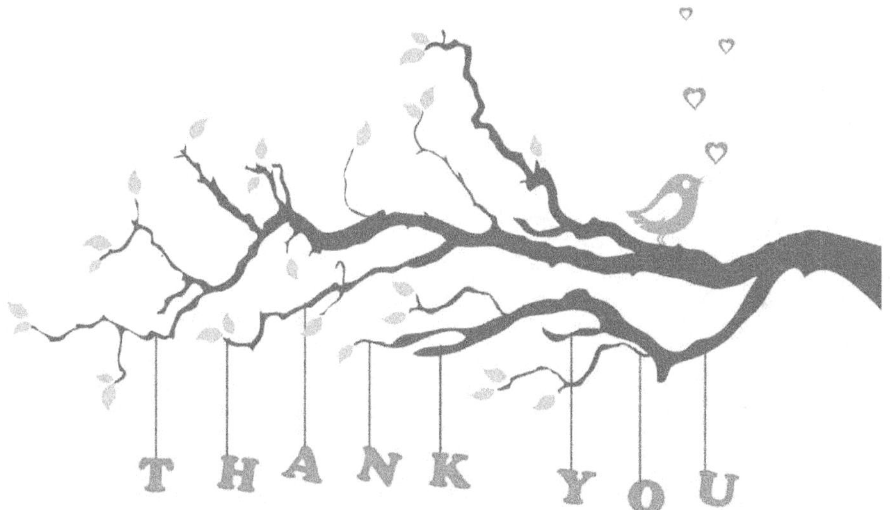

Finally, I want to thank you for reading my book. If you enjoyed the book, please share your thoughts and post a review on the book retailer's website. It would be greatly appreciated!

Best wishes,

Catalina Morris